Pilates for beginners:

Workout routines to change your Body

Table Of Contents

Copyright

Introduction

I want to thank you and congratulate you for downloading the book, *"Pilates for beginners: Workout routines to change your Body."*

This book contains proven steps and strategies how to start having a fit and healthy through easy-to-follow Pilates workout routines.

Pilates is one of the most popular forms of exercise, which was developed by Joseph Pilates. It focuses on the development of the body based on core strength, awareness, and flexibility so as to support graceful movements.

The Pilates method is primarily focused on the improvement of core strength and flexibility. The outcome that you can obtain from doing these Pilates exercises for beginners can be life-changing. This is because you will gain control and balance while strengthening your body. In addition, the exercises can also relax your mind as you move freely. These Pilates exercises can be refreshing especially if you have tried other fitness methods and failed.

It is necessary to learn carrying out Pilates exercise with the proper form, movement, and concentration in order to maximize the method. Some Pilates moves require time in order to be proficient. However, you need not hurry. Take your time until your develop the right form and concentration for carrying out the exercises.

In order to achieve the best results from the fundamental exercises discussed above, you need to learn how to integrate the exercises that you perform. This way, you will be able to emphasize on all your muscles. If you keep doing the same routine, it is more likely that you only cover some of your muscles than all of them. However, if you know the exercises to mix and match, all your muscles will get accustomed to the exercises, prompting you to level up.

The key to progress using the Pilates method is change. Changing your routine shocks your system through new motions; thus, your muscles are constantly challenged to flourish and grow in healthier ways.

Thanks again for downloading this book, I hope you enjoy it!

Chapter 1: History of Pilates

In the last 10 years, Pilates has become a popular workout routine not only among the elite class but also in the fitness mainstream. However, you might ask when and where Pilates began.

In 1912, Joseph Pilates, founder of the Pilates method went to England and worked as a self-defense instructor for detectives. During World War I, he became an "enemy alien" intern among other German nationals. At this time, Joseph created alternatives for his exercises, which he used as a self-defense instructor, sharing them with other internees. Joseph rigged out springs to hospital beds in order for bedridden patients to move their bodies against resistance. This became his first innovation and basis for his equipment designs. In 1918, an influenza epidemic hit England where thousands of people died. However, Joseph's trainees remained strong and resistant against the epidemic and none of them died. Thus, Joseph claimed the efficiency of his system.

When Joseph was released from his internship, he returned to Germany and continued with his method of exercise. The dance community favored Joseph's exercise routine until it became widely known in Germany. However, Joseph left Germany for good when German officials asked him to impart his exercise system to the German army.

In 1926, Joseph immigrated to the United States and later married, Clara. Together, they opened their first fitness studio in New York. During the early 1960s, their clients where innumerable making the Pilates Method popular not only in New York but in other places as well.

In 1964, the Pilates Method made it to the New York Herald Tribune where it was referred to as "pilates" with a small P. The newspaper claimed that young students gather daily in dance classes in the United States to learn the "pilates."

In 1967, Joseph passed away without leaving a will. This meant that he did not designate a line of succession for his Pilates Method. However, Clara continued the operation of the Pilates Studio in New York along with Romana Kryzanowska. In 1970, the latter became the director of the studio after studying the work of Joseph in Peru for 15 years.

Meanwhile, a number of Joseph and Clara's students opened their own Pilates studios in different parts of the United States and other parts of the world including Puerto Rico and New Mexico. This marked the global popularity of the Pilates Method, making it one of the most efficient workout routines today.

The exercises that Joseph Pilates created were primarily to trim and tone the body using a mat. As time passed, Joseph Pilates discovered that he could create variations that adapted to one's own fitness level. This was the start of a successful and proficient exercise program.

Chapter 2: Principles of Pilates

More often than not, Pilates workout routines for beginners help you build an efficient groundwork for Pilates method. The first 30 days of a Pilates routine for beginners is crucial for transforming your life as this period will involve learning what to do and how to move using the principles of Pilates.

The core principles of Pilates give emphasis on centering, controlling, concentrating, developing precision, breathing, and flowing. These principles allow you to be healthy not only physically but mentally as well.

To help you understand Pilates, it is helpful to know its basic principles including concentration, centering, control, and precision.

- Concentration – With the proper focus on the mind body awareness, Pilates believes on establishing an essential connection with your body while obtaining benefits from workout routines. Pilates exercises should be done in slow and precise manner instead of doing them with improper alignment or form. If you want to obtain the maximum benefits of Pilates, your complete concentration is need while performing each exercise.

- Centering – This entails that paying attention to the abdominal muscles or core will make all your other muscles develop and function better. In each Pilates movement, the first area to center you mind is also the center of the body, which is the abdomen.

- Control – Quality is more important in Pilates than quantity. It is better to have control over all your movements than become sloppy. It is also important to repeat each movement regularly to be able to do the exercises correctly. All movements are controlled by the muscles. Thus, by having better control, your movements will shift subtly with greater results.

- Precision – This is another significant factor in Pilates. Precision can be obtained by being aware throughout every movement. Proper form is important in order to obtain optimal benefits from each exercise.

The first day of a Pilates workout routine for beginners is usually the most difficult. This is because you need to learn the fundamental movements that you need to carry out for the rest of your Pilates experience.

During day 1, you need to begin with the basic Pilates movements, which are simple exercises yet significant in building a good form of Pilates routine.

Week 1 begins with day 2 and ends at day 7. This week aims to polish everything that has been learned and carried out during the first day of the routine. Within this week, you should be able to continue the basic Pilates movements and the Pilates routine for beginners.

Week 2 involves carrying out warm up exercises using basic Pilates movements. However, some other exercises are added including, cat/cow back stretch, arms reach and pull, and pelvic curl. During this week, you should be able to move on to the Pilates routine for beginners with side kick exercise series.

Week 3 involves carrying out warm up exercises with basic Pilates movements with additional exercises including saw, side kick series, Pilates push up, swan prep, and leg pull front.

Finally, Week 4 is a repetition of Week 3 only you need to add 10 exercises including single straight leg stretch, crisscross, swan with neck roll, tease with one leg, leg pull front, Pilates push up, double leg lower lift, saw, side kick series, swimming, and seal.

Make time to carry out your Pilates workout routine regularly for a healthier body. Pilates not only helps you look good physically but can also make you function more efficiently.

3: Benefits of Pilates

One of the most significant benefits of Pilates is developing a strong core. Pilates emphasizes on making the abdominal muscles, back, and but stronger. This leads to improved pelvic stability. More so, you will no longer be prone to back injuries.

Another benefit of Pilates is having an improved posture. If you are suffering from a "hunched" back, Pilates allows you to achieve the proper posture by lengthening your neck. The exercises in Pilates help in aligning your posture better and make you sit and stand taller and straighter.

Increased flexibility and strength is another important benefit that Pilates can provide you. Once you start doing Pilates exercises, you also stretch and strengthen your muscles. Thus, your joints have greater motion range.

If you are conscious about the appearance of your body, Pilates can provide you with longer and leaner muscles. These days, many workout routines include Pilates exercises that focus on all the muscles instead of just one body part. Pilates works throughout the body, elongating your muscles while your move with control and precision.

The focus of the first round of this Pilates workout routine is on the abdominal muscles. You might also notice that the exercises included in this round also affect your hip flexors and quadriceps.

The movements in the first round are done from the imprint position, also known as the footprint. The imprint position does not make use of movements in the abdominals. The imprint position prepares the abdominals to control and hold a position while your stomach is continuously pulled in. This position will make you appear you have a smaller waist line.

The second round of this Pilates workout routine focuses on the lower back as well as the thighs, shoulders, and butt. Naturally, you cannot achieve having a flat abs without having a strong back.

The third round of this Pilates workout routine for beginners focuses on the obliques, thighs, and other core muscles. It helps in developing balance and body control. When doing these exercises, make sure that your body is always in a straight line with your hips parallel to the surface. Your legs should try to swing forward, hips tipped back so your abdominal muscles take control.

Why Pilates?

You may be asking yourself why you should practice Pilates versus any other exercise routine such as yoga. The first reason you should give Pilates a try is that it is great for you, many people report seeing results in as little as six weeks. Pilates helps to relieve stress as well as refresh the body and relieve muscle strain.

Pilates helps to with concentration, if you are suffering from attention problems or struggling to maintain focus you will benefit greatly from incorporating Pilates into your life. If you do Pilates correctly you will be able to create a larger range of motion, flexibility and increase your circulation as well as oxygen flow to your organs, tissue and glands.

Pilates is great for those who are not able to do high impact aerobics because the movements are slow and focused. Pilates is also time saving. Where you would have to do an hour of aerobics each day you can start out with 10 minutes of Pilates each day. There are great videos available online absolutely free for beginners. There are also many sites that have entire programs set out for months of Pilates, they start you off doing 10 minutes a day, providing instructive videos until you are able to do one hour per day.

Pilates is also very gentle on your joints so instead of spending an hour on the treadmill and hurting afterward, Pilates can actually help heal your joints. Speaking of healing when you use Pilates, you are able to heal faster as well as recover faster when you are sick.

Pilates is great for your mental health as well. You will feel an overall sense of well-being when you practice Pilates, it helps to reduce symptoms of depression, raise self-esteem, increase will power develop discipline and it increases energy.

Not only can you lose weight by using Pilates but you will find that in just a few weeks you are more flexible and stronger than you have ever been in your life.

Pilates is great for the young and old alike so if you want to make a change in your life no matter what your age all it takes is a few weeks and you will be hooked. After as few as 30 days your life will be changed forever.

Tips And Warnings

1. The first tip is that you need to make time for Pilates every day. This is one reason it is important that you start off small with about 10 minutes per day of working out. Often times when people decide that they want to start a new exercise program, they tend to try and change a lot of different things in their lives. It is important that you only make one change at a time. You should choose to add Pilates into your life, and change nothing else for 30 days. When you try to make too many changes at one time it becomes overwhelming and people give up. So schedule 10 minutes each morning for your Pilates workout, stick with this for 30 days before you make any other changes in your life. This does not include changing your diet which we will talk about later.

2. Be realistic about your goals, this is another reason may people give up, they set the bar too high. How often have you heard someone say they are going to exercise for an hour per day and three days later they have given up. This is why you want to start small. If you are not able to workout for 10 minutes when you start out, start with five minutes. Don't start out trying to do more than 10 minutes per day during the first week. The second week you can add 5 more minutes and so on until you reach an hour per day.

3. Don't push your body too hard. One of the great things with Pilates is that the idea of no pain no gain has no place in it. You will be surprised on your first day when

you don't break a sweat and your muscles are not aching. You will be a little sore the next day but if you are feeling pain you are not doing the exercises correctly check your posture before exercising more.

4. Be patient and exercise regularly. Often times, people will give up after starting because they are expecting some overnight miracle. This never happens, therefore they quit without seeing results. If you want to see results when you use Pilates, you need to be consistent as well as patient. Although Pilates is one of the fastest ways I have ever seen to produce results often times people get upset because they are not losing weight right away. Sometimes you may see that you begin gaining a little weight before you see any loss the reason for this is that you are building your core muscles, don't get upset, you will see results.

5. Speeding up the Pilates exercises will not make Pilates more effective. Pilates is meant to be slow if you speed up the exercises thinking you are going to get a more effective workout you are mistaken. Do the Pilates exercises the way they are designed to be done.

6. Many times people do not hold the correct posture when they are doing Pilates exercises, this will cause strain on your body. For example, many exercises have you holding your head off of the floor, sometimes people will gaze at the ceiling jutting their chin out away from their body, this will cause strain on your neck. Instead you should hold your chin near to your chest as if you are holding a piece of fruit in place. Make sure you are not pressing your chin hard against your

chest like you are trying to juice the fruit, this will cause strain and often headache.

7. Make sure you are not spacing out when you are doing Pilates. This is very easy to do but you need to remember that Pilates is about brining your mind and body into balance, in order to do this you need to keep your mind focused while you are working out. If you create mental images of what is going on in your body, it will help greatly with your focus.

8. Make sure you are contracting your abs while you are in each position, at first this is not as important as you learn the exercises but this will help to build your core strength, it is also great to help with focus. If you are focusing on your abdominals while you are exercising your mind will not wonder.

9. Make sure when you start out that you are using programs, videos or DVD's that focus on beginners. You don't want to try exercises that you are not ready for and end up hurting yourself.

10. Point those toes, if you find that an exercise is difficult for you remember that pointing your toes can make it easier, this is one reason Pilates is such a great compliment to ballet.

11. For best results do Pilates two to four times per week. Exercising once per week is not going to cut it and if you exercise more than every other day you will get very sore and likely give up exercising.

12. Do Pilates on an empty stomach, or at earliest, two hours after eating. You should try to make sure your

bladder is empty as well, this will make it easier to contract your abs while you are exercising.

13. If you have trouble sleeping Pilates will help.

14. When you are working out you need to make sure you have the correct clothing on. Yoga pants and a t-shirt work great, shorts are not recommended for Pilates because they tend to be very uncomfortable when you are completing full range of motion leg exercises. If you do not want to wear yoga pants, you should dress comfortably and wear loose clothes that will allow you to move your body freely and easily.

15. Keep a small towel handy that you can roll up. You can place this under your head to prevent straining or under your hips when you are lying on your stomach to prevent pressure on your hip bones. Do not place the towel under your neck this will cause your bones to be out of alinement. Make sure you only use the towel under your neck.

16. If you are trying to lose weight with Pilates, you have to have a sensible diet, just exercising is not going to do anything for you if you do not eat right we will talk about diet later on in the book.

17. Make sure you take the time to warm up your muscles before doing Pilates, in the next section I will go over Pilates warm up exercises.

Pilates Warm Up Exercises

Warming up before doing Pilates and cooling down after Pilates exercises is essential to your work out. It helps prevent muscle strain, helps your mind transition in to working out mode and then back into normal life. Warming up will also increase blood flow to all of your muscles preparing them for the workout, it will help to ensure you do not become out of breath to easily, it will allow your heart rate to raise slowly instead of having a rapid increase of blood pressure.

You should warm up before each session of Pilates for at least five to ten minutes, you will have to spend more time warming up for very intense work outs and about five minutes for low intensity work outs. All you really need to do is get your body ready for exercise.

The first warm up exercise I want to teach you is called the shoulder roll. You want to start sitting with your legs crossed, allow your hands to relax on your knees, inhale as you begin to roll your shoulders back exhaling when you complete the circle. Repeat this exercise three times and when you have finished, repeat the same process except this time roll your shoulders forward. Repeat the front shoulder roll three times.

Next you will stretch your legs out in front of you, breathing naturally you will circle your feet in one direction three times, then in the reverse direction three more times. Point your toes, hold for 3 seconds and then pull them back toward you, repeat this five times.

Now you are going to lie down on your back with your knees bent, while keeping your pelvis stable you are going to rotate your leg out, straighten the leg out and then draw it back into the starting position. Repeat this four times and then switch to the other leg.

For the final warm up exercise you should lay on your side, raise one leg up to create a 90 degree angle with your legs, stretch your free are out in front of you and then keeping your eyes on your arm raise it to become parallel with the raised leg. Inhaling as you raise your arm exhale and lower both the arm and the leg back to the starting position. Repeat this four times and then switch sides.

That is all you have to do to warm up before your Pilates session, you can use the same exercises to cool down or if you are using a video or DVD you can follow what the instructor has you do. I strongly suggest that you do not try to do Pilates without some help. It is best if you can have an instructor but I understand that is not always possible. Finding DVD's for beginners or videos online is the next best thing this way you will be able to see what your body should look like when you are completing each of these moves.

Breathing is very important when it comes to Pilates so it is also good to have a video or DVD to help instruct you on when to breath and how to breath. It is very difficult to learn breathing techniques simply by reading a book, you need someone to tell you how and when to breathe. This is not to say that you will not see benefits of Pilates if you do not have a video that can teach you the breathing techniques because you will see some. This is simply saying that you will not see the results you could if you took some time to look up the breathing techniques. These can be found absolutely free online and if you work through free Pilates programs you can find online, you will be instructed in the videos about breathing.

4: How to Get Started

Pilates is a non-complex type of exercise with a balanced system that suits novices, experts, and even elite athletes. It offers great results irrespective of fitness level or age. Pilates is a tried and tested method that enhances one's health and wellness. Thus, it is more than just a fitness trend.

Pilates is different from spinning class or aerobics given that you cannot jump from one level to another without mastering the former. In Pilates, it is important to master each basic exercise prior to taking advanced levels.

On the other hand, more than just teaching the fundamentals, basic Pilates exercises.

Pilates is considered a powerful method, which are also used by many sports enthusiasts, athletes, and dance experts. Many successful fitness professionals include Pilates movements in the daily or regular exercise programs.

Pilates exercises can be performed by people of various fitness levels. Even individuals who are overweight or out of shape can adapt to the simple yet efficient Pilates movements. It is also an ideal fitness method for athletes because the movements are not stressful both to the mind and body.

In addition, Pilates exercises are ideal for all ages. Most senior citizens love to carry out Pilates exercises because of their low impact. The exercises are not prone to hurt the ligaments or cause injuries.

More often than not, getting into fitness workouts are challenging and exciting at the same time specifically if you are serious about seeing changes in your body. There are many fitness programs available today including running, Zumba, and yoga among others. On the other hand, Pilates is considered the most efficient among all fitness and wellness programs today.

Once you decide to perform Pilates exercises, you need to understand what it would take to accomplish every movement. Unlike other fitness programs that primarily focus on general physique, Pilates emphasizes on making your core strong and working efficiently through the rest of the body.

The key to a proper and efficient Pilates workout routine is proper breathing, pacing, rhythm. You have to keep your mind one with your body.

Ultimately, you can be assured of progress in your well-being regardless if you are a beginner or advanced performer of Pilates exercises.

When you start with Pilates you need to make sure no matter what your fitness level is that you start with at a beginners level. If you try to jump past the beginners level you are going to miss out on vital information that you will need later on.

You may also subject yourself to injury because you did not take the time to learn everything at a beginners level.

If you want to get started with Pilates, congratulations this book is the first step but I hate to break it to you, no book is going to teach you everything you need to know about Pilates what you will have to do is actually start practicing.

Of course it is very simple to figure out how to get started with Pilates at a gym, sign up for the class and follow the directions you are given. So for this next section I am going to focus more on what you need to do if you want to get started using Pilates at home.

The first thing you are going to have to do is to choose an area where you will be able to work out. Some people may choose to do this in the living room where they will be able to watch DVD's on a television but personally I do not like the entire DVD route. I instead take my laptop to my designated work out area which is a large open space in the entrance of my home. This is where I can play the videos and my entire family is able to workout all together. Where ever you choose, make sure it is an area where you will not be distracted or disturbed. Make sure your pets are kept out of the area as well especially if you have larger dogs, they are great for knocking you over or interfering with your concentration while you are exercising. When you choose your area make sure you have plenty of space to extend your arms and legs completely. You will not receive the benefits of Pilates if you are unable to do the exercises correctly.

The next thing you are going to have to do is purchase a few small items. You can go out and purchase a Pilates mat or order one online, I cannot tell you exactly which one to order because it all depends on the surface you want to be working on. You can also just use a towel if you don't want to purchase a mat when you are just starting out.

Next you will need to choose your Pilates videos. Like I said earlier, some people choose to use DVD's but I would much rather use videos I can find online, the reason for this is because if I have a question I cannot ask it to the people who are on the DVD's, online videos especially if they come from fitness groups provide more support when it comes to you having questions or needing a bit of help. Most of these people who post these videos or create the blogs with videos in them are Pilates instructors and they understand there are just some people who are not going to go to the gym or pay a private instructor. All you have to do is ask them your question and they respond fairly quickly. But if you choose to use DVD's at this point you will need to decide which DVD you will use and purchase it. If you choose to use online videos you will need to find those and bookmark them.

Then you want to take all of your measurements. You want to know how much you weigh, what the measurements of your waist, hips and chest are. You can take this further by measuring your thighs, arms, neck and so forth. Finally you need to find out what your BMI is, most doctors can give you this or you can have it calculated online for free. You will want to write these down because in 30 days you are going to check them again to see what your results are.

Now this is going to work one of two ways. If you are using Pilates to lose weight you are going to see your numbers go down. If you are using Pilates as a way to strength train you want to make sure your numbers are only going up except for your BMI. Make sure that stays at an acceptable level.

You are not going to weigh your compare your measurements until the first 30 days is completed.

Lastly you will want to create a plan. There are tons of websites out there that offer free Pilates plans for beginners. If you want to create your own calendar that is great as well. This is what a week looks like for me:

Monday- Full body work out.

Tuesday- 10 sit ups, ab work out and 10 minute ab sculpt

Wednesday- 30 second planks, butt work out, total body Pilates.

Thursday- Cardio warm up and inner thigh work out

Friday- Total body work out followed by abs and butt work out.

Saturday- 15 crunches, cardio warm up, arm work out

Sunday – is my off day where I make sure I get enough protein. (We will talk about diet later)

As you can see I do not work the same muscle groups two days in a row, this is how I am able to work out 6 days a week instead of 2. This may look like a lot to you reading it but really it only takes about 30 minutes a day. That is all that I want to spend on working out at this time and it seems to work great for me. You may find that you need less time or more time.

Since all of us are different you can set up your own calendar to help you reach your goals or just download one from the internet.

I like to keep track of my work outs on a separate calendar, actually I have three separate calendars, one for working out, one for bills and appointments and one for work. I find this easier for me. But then of course I also put everything into my online planner to remind me of what I should be doing and when. It is all up to you how you plan everything out to fit in your schedule but I suggest doing your Pilates early in the morning even if this means that you will be getting up earlier. You will have more energy once you have been exercising for a little while and although it may be very difficult to force yourself to get up earlier in the morning to exercise you will see a difference in your energy levels as early as the first week.

DIET

Oh the four lettered word no one wants to hear. It is time to talk about diet. As I stated earlier if you want to use Pilates to lose weight you are going to have to change your diet. This does not have to be done overnight but I do suggest that you plan on changing the way you eat for your next shopping trip. Go ahead and use up the foods you have in your home right now, I do not believe in throwing food away so if you want to get rid of any of the food in your home please donate any unopened foods to your local food pantry. There are people who rely on these donations so please don't just throw it away.

The first thing you are going to have to change is the amount of water you consume. If you want to lose the most weight possible you have to start drinking large amounts of water. You need to make sure you are drinking at least 4 liters or one gallon of water each day. You can use green tea to flavor this water but DO NOT add sugar, you can also use a bit of lemon if you have trouble drinking plain water. One thing I have found with people who just do not like water is that if they put ice in it or cool it in the fridge they are much more likely to drink it.
Drinking this much water usually means you are going to give up pretty much everything else you are drinking. This is a great thing to do, you should give up all soda, sugary drinks and even coffee, black coffee is fine in the morning but not throughout the day because it will dehydrate you and the caffeine will interfere with your sleep.

Drinking more water is going to be one of the easiest things you will change when it comes to losing weigh with Pilates. If you think about it, it really does not require any will power to drink more water, you simply make yourself a cold glass and give your body what it needs.

Often our minds will confuse hunger with thirst so you may find that by simply drinking more water you are not hungry as often as you thought you were. Maintaining hydration will also ensure you keep your metabolism as high as it can be. You see when your body it dehydrated it tends to slow down, your thinking processes slow, you need more sleep and your metabolism slows down causing you to store more fat.

Instead of drinking coffee first thing in the morning, before your work out grab a glass or two of ice cold water this will boost your metabolism as you start your day. The water also helps to lubricate your joints so that you do not experience pain when you are exercising.

I have one warning for you when it comes to drinking water, if it is very hot out and you are sweating a lot make sure you do not drink too much water. Now this may seem a little silly at first but you will be sweating out a lot of your salt, this is what causes people to end up in the hospital, this is also one reason you will see people drink a lot of sports drinks in the summer. I am no advocate of sports drinks because I do not believe in drinking your calories and often they do more harm than good but you do need to keep an eye on your electrolytes. If necessary you can add a bit of salt to your water but don't add too much.

Let's talk about food. Yes you are going to have to give up the fried eggs and bacon, well at least most of the time. I do eat these foods on my off day because I know that no one will stick to anything if they feel deprived. Do I eat them on every off day? No about once a month and I am okay. A great breakfast you can have after your workout is plain yogurt over a few sliced strawberries sprinkled with sunflower seeds and drizzled in just a bit of honey for sweetness.

For lunch you should focus on inexpensive proteins such as tuna, hard boiled eggs and of course make sure you eat at least one fruit and one vegetable. One of my favorite lunches is a half a can of tuna with wheat crackers five baby carrots topped off by a banana and a glass of water.

Salads, soups and other homemade foods are great for dinner. What you have to do is watch your portion sizes. You will still be able to make a cheese burger, use a whole wheat bun, instead of a white bun, have baked sweet potato fries instead of French fries and make sure you use lots of vegetables on your burger. Now you will notice I said A cheese burger, you are going to find that you are eating way more food than you actually need. Eat a cheese burger if you still feel hungry start drinking that water. I often prefer to have a large salad or even homemade soups or stews. The majority of the meal is vegetables, but I also make sure that there is enough protein in the meal as well. Protein is very important when you are working out for building muscles so don't cut the protein in your meals.

For a snack twice a day you can eat a piece of fruit or some vegetables depending on what you want. I want to quickly address a myth that I have come head to head with lately and that is that it is more expensive to eat healthy than it is to buy junk food and I want you to understand that is simply not true. As you probably see you have been eating a lot more than you actually should be eating, when you add exercise and drinking a lot of water in, you will realize you don't need that much food. You will actually be spending a lot less on your meals than you were before plus you will be saving thousands on medical bills in the future.

If you are not ready to make major changes in your diet or you are part of a family that will not be making the same changes as you, simply start watching your portions, cut out the cakes, candies and sugary drinks as well as all of the processed snacks, and you will start to see a difference. When I first started I simply stopped eating off of a dinner plate and started eating off of a saucer, this made a huge difference in the amount of food I was eating.

Now you know exactly what you need to do in order to get started with Pilates. Now you have to make it happen.

5: Basic Exercises of Pilates for Beginners

Neutral Spine

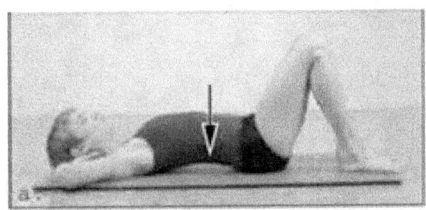
Too much curve (anterior pelvic tilt).

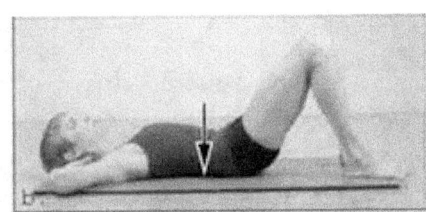
not enough curve (posterior pelvic tilt).

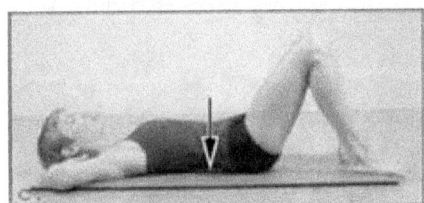
and just right (neutral pelvis).

Prior to carrying out the Pilates workout routine for beginners, it is important that you achieve Neutral Spine. Neutral Spine refers to the optimal posture that one needs to perform all exercises in Pilates correctly. It is a way to activate your muscles properly specifically the transversus abdominis and pelvic floor. The starting position of Pilates involves an exercise that locates the right position of neutral spine by pressing the lower back into the floor; thus, having your back flat on the surface. After which, the spine is released into a small arch. Once you achieve these two points, the 3 curves of the spine should be in their natural position. This then will be the starting position that will guide you throughout the set of Pilates basic workout routine.

The basic move of the neutral spine exercise involves:

1. Pressing down your back in an even surface, usually on a mat, with your arms on your sides. Your knees should be bent while the distance between your legs and feet is hip apart. Your legs and feet should also be parallel to each other.

2. Inhale.
3. Exhale then make use of your abs so that your lower spine is pressed on the surface.

4. Inhale in order to release.

5. Exhale again while pulling the lower spine up in order to create an arch of your low back.

6. Inhale again to release.

The Hundred

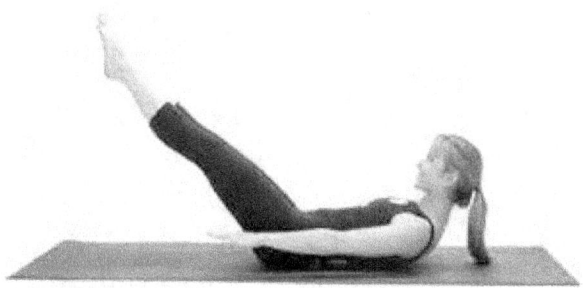

This exercise focuses on breathing and the abdominals. The latter should be pulled deeply using your full lung capability, breathing into your lower ribs and back. The Hundred is one of the most essential moves you should learn in Pilates because it is always included in a warm-up session. This exercise helps in strengthening the core through requiring the abdominals and back muscles to function together. The hundred is probably the most popular Pilates exercise. It focuses on the stomach and the core. It requires added concentration on endurance and breathing. In addition, your legs should be straight up high as you lie flat on the mat with your head constantly down.

The basic move of the hundreds exercise involves:

1. Start by lying flat on your back on the mat. Your shoulders must be held down. Your feet should be pointed and the body should be elongated in such a way that it is stretched with your head top.

2. While your back is flat on the mat, bring your legs up and head off the surface. Make sure that your neck stays on a neutral position while your chin is tucked.

3. Extend your arms and start lifting and lowering them around 2 inches from the mat. Breathe in to lift and exhale to lower your arms.

4. Do the up and down movements 5 times with 10 repetitions until you reach a hundred.

Roll Up

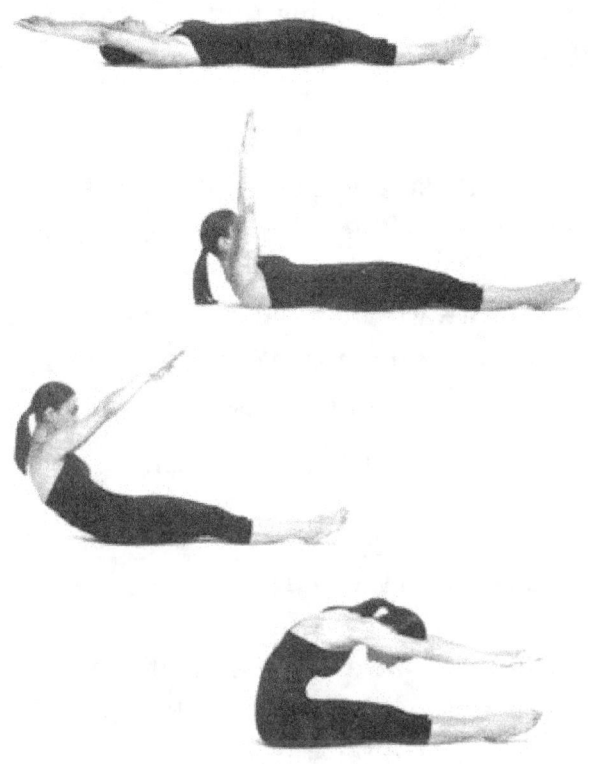

This exercise focuses on the abdominals. In order to roll up and down, you should use your abdominals with sufficient control. Your legs should not be lifted from the mat. The roll up or roll down is also an essential warm-up exercise, which is often included in most Pilates workout routines. This exercise helps in strengthening the abdominal muscles.

The basic move of the roll up exercise involves:

1. Begin by lying on your back, keeping your legs straight and arms stretched above the head. Your shoulders should remain down on the mat.

2. While your back is lying flat on the mat, lift your arms in a slow move toward the ceiling as you inhale.

3. As you exhale, roll forward in a slow motion while trying to lift your spine off the mat. Your head should remain straight while your eyes are focused forward. Your stomach should be tight instead of crunched.

4. Inhale again while stretching over your legs. Exhale as you slowly roll back down on the mat.

5. Make sure not to pause; however, as you inhale, roll up again to start with the second repetition. Perform the movements until you reach 10 repetitions.

One Leg Circle

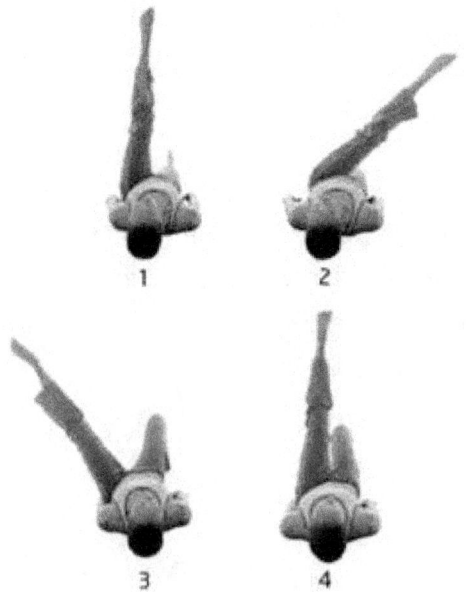

The one leg circle focuses on the pelvis and the hips. This is exercise is also for the thighs, hip flexors, and abdominals. The pelvis should be stable while your leg moves. A Pilates warm-up would not be complete without doing the one-leg circle. This exercise helps in opening up your hips as well as increasing your flexibility.

The basic move of the one leg circle exercise involves:

1. While your arms are on your sides, palms faced down, lie flat on your back. Pull in your abs as you extend your left leg towards the ceiling. Make sure that your toe is pointed.

2. In a clockwise motion, rotate your left leg as if drawing a circle on air. Inhale while you draw the circle from 12 o'clock to 6 o'clock. Exhale from 6 o'clock to 12 o'clock.

   Do the same in the opposite direction.

3. Put down your left leg on the mat and start again this time with your right leg.

This exercise can be optimized in 10 repetitions, 5 times for each leg.

Roll like a Ball

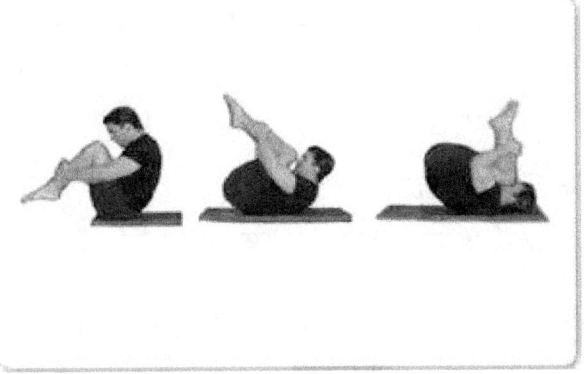

This exercise is focused on the abdominals. You should be in a curved position throughout this exercise. You should be able to roll back using your abs instead of your upper body back.

The basic move of the roll like a ball exercise involves:

1. Start this exercise by sitting on the mat, knees towards your chest. Your arms should be holding your legs.

2. Rock back to keep the mat connected with the base of your tailbone. Bring your feet up slightly off from the mat.

3. Breathe in as your roll back to the back of your shoulder blades.

4. Breathe out as your roll back to the sitting position at the start of the exercise.

One-Leg Stretch

The one-leg stretch is a basic Pilates exercise that makes use of your core strength. You should have sufficient core strength to tone your abs and obliques and carry out alternating leg extensions.

The basic move of the one-leg stretch exercise involves:

1. With your back flat on the surface, put your arms on your sides while your palms are faced down.

2. Raise your head and shoulders off the mat. Hold your right knee while extending out your left leg. The distance between the mat and the raised leg depends on the strength of your abdominals and your leg's weight.

3. Make sure to align your head and bend your elbows. Switch sides in a slow move while you extend your right leg. Inhale for 2 quick counts then exhale for 2 quick counts as well.

This exercise should be done in 10 repetitions, 5 times for each side.

Arms-Over

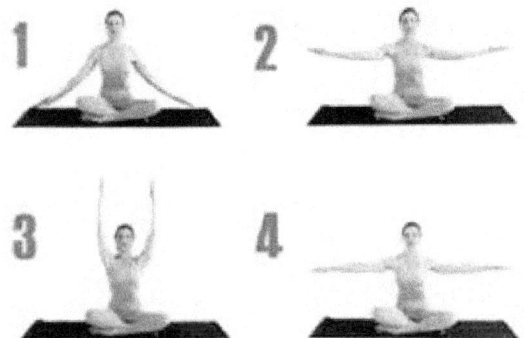

The arms-over exercise is focused on keeping your balance while the torso is forced by moving the arms over your head. Arms-over exercise can increase the range of your motion in your shoulders. It involves inhaling from the start position while raising fingertips to aim for the ceiling; exhaling to bring down the arms; inhaling to bring up arms again; and exhaling to release.

The basic move of the arms-over exercise involves:

1. Beginning with the basic or start position.

2. Inhale as you raise your fingertips seemingly reaching the ceiling.

3. Exhale in order to bring your arms down toward your sides.

4. Inhale while you raise your arms again.

5. Exhale to release arms to the surface.

Pelvic Clock

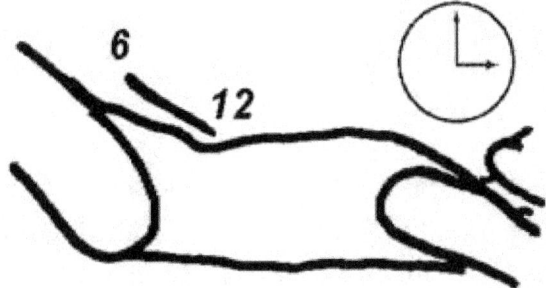

This exercise involves imagining a clock placed flat on the abdomen with the 12 exactly at the bellybutton, 3 on the left hip, 6 on the pubic bone, and 9 on the right hip; starting and controlling movements using abdominal muscles; moving around the clock with the 12 pulled down first followed by 3, 6, and 9. The pelvic clock is a Pilates workout routine that increases your knowledge on the correct pelvic position. It helps strengthen your muscles required for the stability of your pelvis.

The basic move of the pelvic clock exercise involves:

1. Picturing a clock placed flat on the lower abs. The 12 in the clock should be in your bellybutton while the 3 should be on your left hip. The 6 in the clock should be on your pubic bone while the 9 should be on your right hip.

2. Move around the clock sequentially by pulling the 12 down using your abdominal muscles. This will start and control the entire movement.

3. Rotate the 3, 6, and 9.

Although the movements in the pelvic clock exercise are small, your focus should be on moving your pelvis without affecting the stability of your body. Your hips should not rise from the surface.

Knee Folds

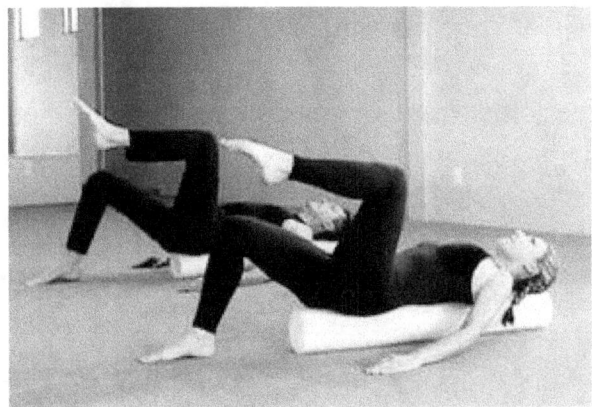

This exercise involves inhaling from the start position while feeling the abdominal muscles to contract; lifting a leg to be in a deep-fold position to the hip; exhaling to return foot on the floor with abdominal control. The primary goal of the knee folds exercise is to move your leg in the hip socket without affecting the stability of your pelvis. This exercise is significant in most movements that you do every day including walking, lifting, and sitting.

The basic move of the knee folds exercise involves:

1. Beginning with the basic or start position.

2. Inhale while feeling your abdominal muscles as you lift a leg. The leg should be able to bend deep at the hip.

3. Exhale and put down your leg making sure that you maintain abdominal control. Make sure that your thigh does not take over your movements.

When doing the knee folds exercise, make sure your hip does not go up with the leg. You need to keep your tailbone flat on the surface.

Angel Arms

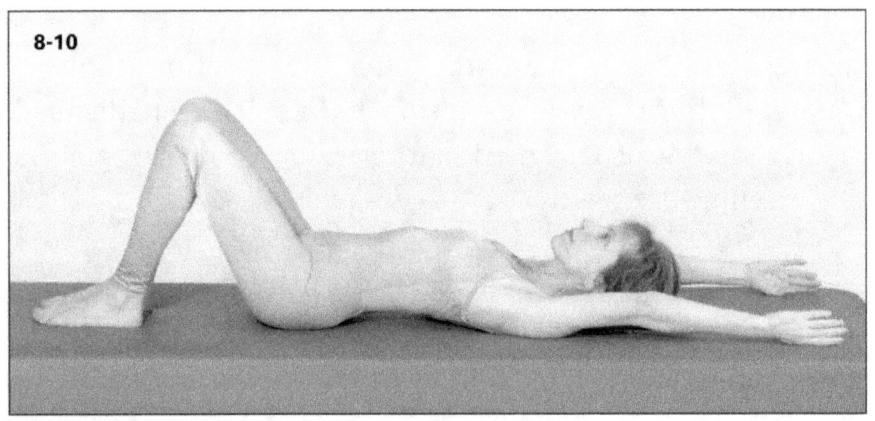

8-10

Angel arms exercise is quite similar to arms-over where different muscles are engaged in the routine. Angel arms exercise helps increase your knowledge on using your arms and shoulders without affecting the alignment of your ribs and back.

The basic move in the angel arms exercise involves:

1. Beginning with the basic or start position.

2. Inhale as your arms sweep out to your sides along the surface.

3. Exhale in order to return your arms on your sides.

4. Like in the arms-over exercise, make sure your abs stay engaged when doing the angel arms routine. The ribs should stay down while the shoulders should remain down as you raise your arms.

Head Nod

Head nod exercise is one of the integral parts of most Pilates workout routines. It is an extension of the spine's lengthening. The head nod is usually used in forward bends of the spine as well as rolling exercises.

The basic move in the head nod exercise involves:

1. Beginning with the basic or start position

2. Inhale in order to lengthen the spine while tilting down your chin towards your chest. The head should stay on the surface.

3. Exhale in order to return to the start position.

4. Inhale in order to tip your head back.

5. Exhale in order to return to the start position.

Kneeling Rear Leg Raises

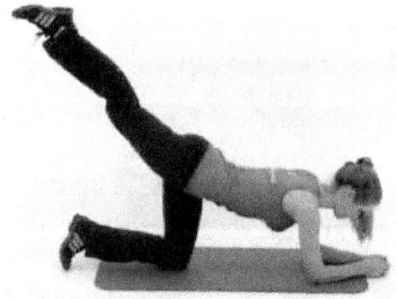

The Pilates kneeling rear leg raises can be executed in 15 seconds for each leg.

The basic move in the kneeling rear leg raises exercise involves:

1. First, you have to get down on your knees with a balanced weight between the elbows and knees. Your knees should be positioned right under your hip joints while your elbows should be under the sockets of your shoulder. Your core muscles should be engaged through pulling your belly button to your spine.

2. Next, one of your legs should be extended back with your toes pointed to the ground without touching the surface. Keep your leg straight and your hips stationary.

3. Then, lift your leg to the highest point that you can without bending or arching your back. Lower your leg slowly at least an inch from the ground. Make sure that your leg does not touch the ground until you are done with the repetitions.

4. Do each step to the other leg.

Side Plank with Leg Raises

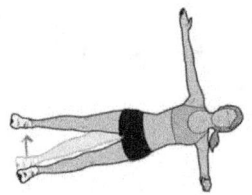

The Pilates side plank with leg raises can also be executed in 15 seconds.

The basic move in the side plank with leg raises exercise involves:

1. The first step to doing this exercise is to lie on your right side making sure that your right knee is bent at 90° and your left leg is extended. Support your upper body on your forearm and elbow while you press your shoulder down. Then, inhale.

2. Next, exhale while lifting your hips so your body would be in a straight line from your head to your knee.

3. Your left hand should then be placed on your hip while keeping the straight line from both your shoulders perpendicularly with the ground. Then, inhale.

4. Exhale as you raise your left leg to the highest point that you can and inhale while you lower your leg back slightly away from the ground.

5. Repeat on the opposite side when all repetitions are done.

Back Bows

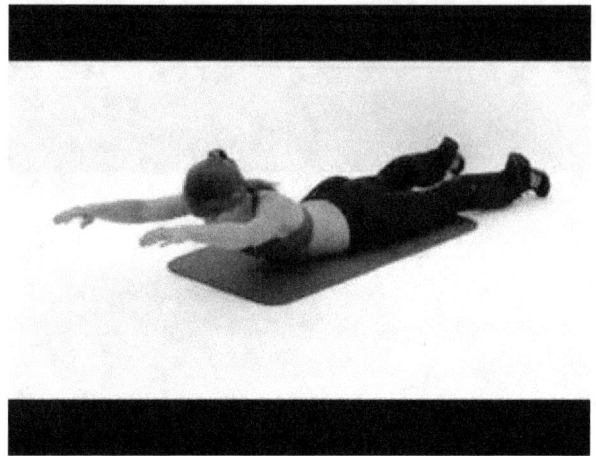

In 15 minutes, you can execute the Pilates back bows.

The basic move in the back bows exercise involves:

1. First, you need to lie face down on the mat while your arms should be above your head.

2. Inhale and contract your core and legs. Exhale as you raise your arms, chest, and legs off the ground to the highest point that you can reach. Your arms and legs should be straight.

3. Inhale and lower down slowly to the ground with your arms, chest, and legs slightly touching the ground prior to repeating the movement.

Make sure to continue and not let your core relax until all repetitions have been down.

Table Tops

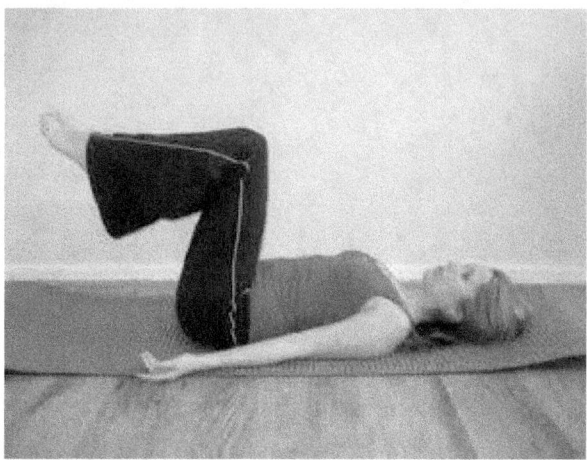

In 15 seconds for each leg, the Pilates table tops can be executed.

The basic move in the table tops exercise involves:

1. Lie on the mat as your feet stay on the ground and your knees at 90° angle. Then, inhale.

2. Exhale slowly as you move to the imprint position. Slowly inhale as you bring one leg off the ground. Make sure your knee is kept at a 90° angle.

3. Pause once your knee is positioned directly over the hip joint.

4. Exhale as you lower your foot back to the mat. Your knee should still stay at 90° angle. Once your foot touches the mat, relax your leg. Inhale slowly as your raise the other leg to the same position prior to exhaling and lowering the leg.

Alternate the legs and relax both, allowing your core to relax.

Chapter 6: Other Popular Pilates Exercises

- Pilates Warm-Up Exercises – These are moves that will teach you the basic Pilates movements while preparing your body to carry out more complicated exercises as you move on to the harder levels.

- Chest Lift – The focus of this exercise is the abdominal muscles specifically the upper abs. Although it may seem like a crunch, the abdominals should be pulled down into a deep scoop while control a smooth curl upwards and roll down.

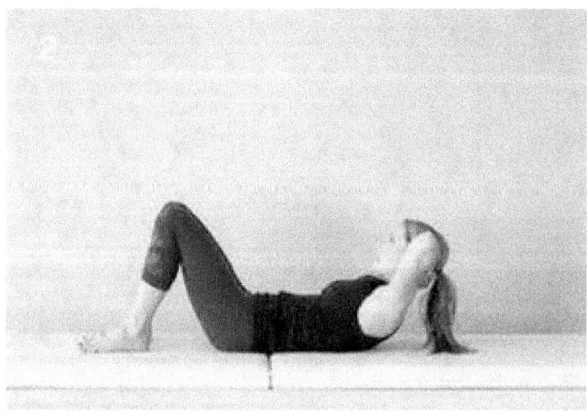

- Open Leg Balance – This exercise focuses on the hamstring and abdominals. As much as possible, keep your balance through abdominal control instead of pulling your legs on.

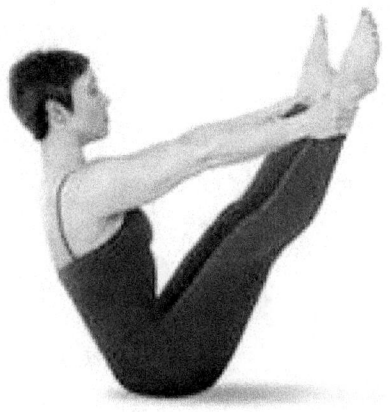

- Side Kick Series – This exercise focuses on all thigh muscles and abdominals. Your ribs should be lifted throughout the exercise and not sinking them to your mat.

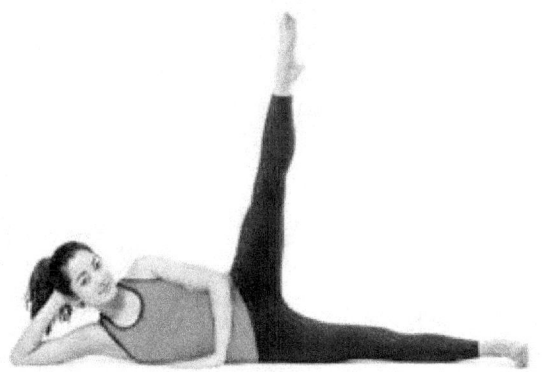

- Front Plank – This exercise is for the shoulders, arms, back extensors, and abdominals. You should be able to hold in a line from your heel to ears. Engage and squeeze together your leg and bones for sitting.

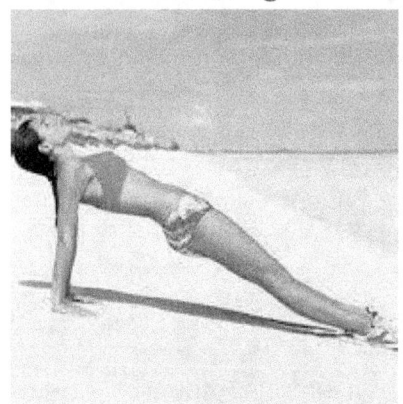

- Saw – This exercise is for the inner thigh, hamstrings, back, and oblique abdominals. Make sure that your hips are anchored and leveled while turn to the side. You should be able to extend your back arm when reaching forward.

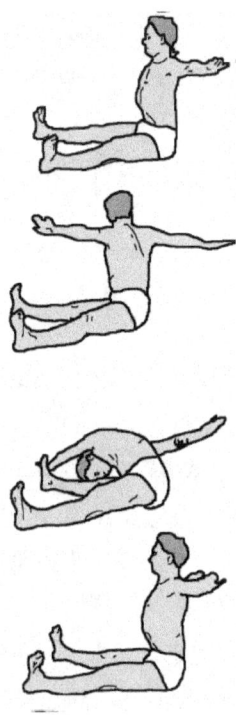

- Mermaid – This exercise focuses on side stretching. Your body should be flat when you stretch sideways like you are positioned between two glass sheets.

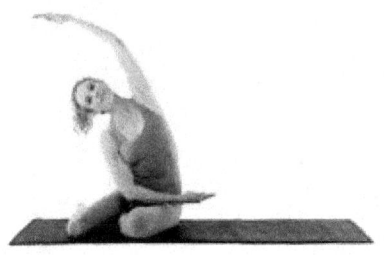

- Swan Prep – This exercise focuses on abdominal stretch and back extensors. It is a counter stretch to most forward flexion routines in Pilates.

- Wall Roll Down – This exercise focuses on the hamstring and back stretch. It is used as a transition move for good posture in daily living.

- Toe Dip – This exercise starts with your back flat on the mat while keeping your legs bent at 90 degrees. Your thighs should be straight up and calves parallel to the surface. Hands should rest on your sides, palms down. Your abs should be contracted while your lower back is pressed towards the floor. Inhale as you lower your left leg in 2 counts. You should only move from your hip as you dip your toes toward the mat without touching it. Exhale and raise your leg in 2 counts to the start position. Repeat movements with your right leg. Make sure to alternate between your legs until reaching 12 repetitions for each.

- Leg Kick – Lie on your left side while your legs are kept straight together, forming one long line. You should be
able to lift your ribs from the mat as you prop up on your left forearm and elbow. Your head should face towards the ceiling. Place your right hand on the mat to maintain your balance. Raise your right leg, hip level and flex your foot while your toes are

pointed forward. Exhale while kicking and swinging your right leg forward as far as you can for 2 quick counts. Inhale while pointing your toes. Swing leg back past the left leg. Do this in 6 repetitions without putting down your leg. Switch to your other side and repeat movements.

- Cat Stretch – Inhale to prepare for this exercise. As you exhale, focus on flattening your abdominals by imagining your belly button being pulled gently towards your spine. Your abdominal muscles should be pulled in while you form a small curve on your lower, middle, and upper back. Inhale and stay for a while in this position. Reverse the movement as you begin to exhale. Make sure that you keep your neck, upper, middle, and lower backs straight as you return to the neutral position. Keep your abdominals contracted. Repeat the movement 4 times.

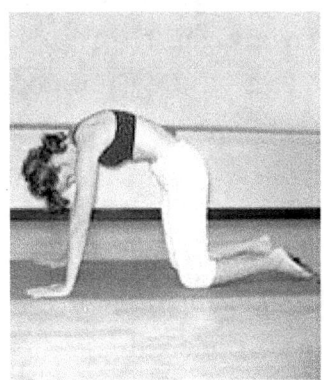

- Opposite Arm and Leg Reaches – Begin this exercise by inhaling. As you exhale, lift your right hand and left knee from the mat. Make sure they are both extended in opposite directions. Inhale to return to the start position then exhale. Do this movement 6 times, 3 times for each side.

- Upper Back Extension – Inhale as you prepare for the exercise. Exhale while keeping your shoulders down on the mat. Your neck should be in line and extended up from the mat. Inhale and stay in this position while imagine extending forwards from your head. Exhale and return your back to the mat. Repeat this movement 4 times while maintaining control of your abdominals.

- Jumping Oblique Twist – Start this exercise by standing, feet together. Raise your arms to shoulder height, hands in front of the chest. Simultaneously hop and twist as your feet lands pointed to your left. Keep your chest forward. Repeat movement with your feet landing pointed to your right.

- Russian Twist – Start by sitting, knees bent and heels on the mat. Allow your torso to tilt back slightly while engaging your abs and creating a small arch on your chest towards the ceiling. Your back should be flat and spine straight. Keep your arms in front of your chest as you twist your torso.

Rotate shoulders as far as you can to the left and

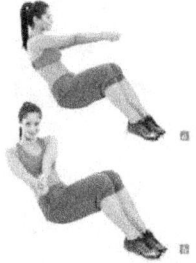

right.

- Windshield Wipers – Lie flat on your back, arms on your sides, palms down. Your thighs should be parallel to the surface while you bend your knees at a 90-degree angle. Simultaneously rotate your hips and thighs to the left as far as you can while keeping your shoulders down to the mat. In a slow motion, bring your hips and thighs back to the center. Repeat movement rotating to the right.

- Heel Slides - This exercise begins by lying on your back. Your hands should stay on your sides in neutral spine position. Keep your transversus abdominis and pelvic floor muscles engaged until you finish the exercise. Next, straighten one knee in a slow motion and return to the start position. Make sure to keep your pelvis and spine steady as you breathe normally. This exercise should be carried out 10 times alternating between your legs.

- Leg Openings – Start this exercise with your back flat on the surface. Hands should be on your sides in neutral spine position. Just like in the first exercise, keep your pelvic floor muscles and transversus abdominis engaged throughout the exercise. Then, take one knee to the side in slow motion and return to the start position. Breathe normally as you keep your pelvis and spine steady. Repeat the movement 10 times alternating between your legs.

- Leg Lifts – Begin this exercise by lying on your back. Hands should be by your sides in neutral spine position. Keep your pelvic floor muscles and transversus abdominis activated at all times. Lift one leg slowly and return to start position. Again, your pelvis and spine should not move. Breathe normally. This exercise should be repeated 10 times alternating between your legs.

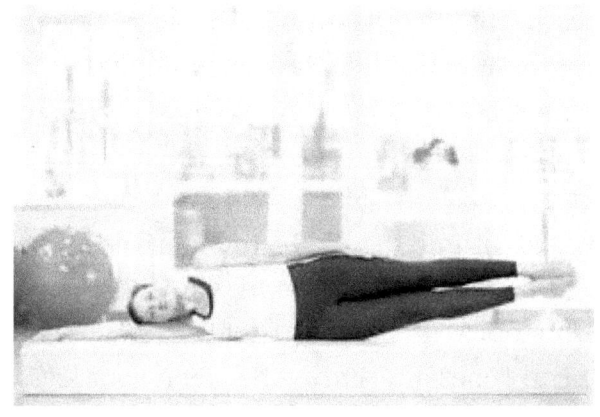

- Heel Taps – This exercise begins with lying on your back in neutral spine position. Hands should be on your sides while your hips and knees are bent on a 90degree angle. Keep your transversus abdominis and pelvic floor muscles engaged until done with the exercise. Lower one leg slowly until your heel reaches the floor. Return to the start position. Always keep your pelvis and spine steady as you breathe normally. This exercise should be performed 10 times alternating between your legs.

- Bridging – As with the previous exercises, lie on your back in neutral spine position when you start this exercise. Keep your pelvic floor muscles and transversus abdominis engaged until you finish the exercise. Lift your bottom slowly, pushing toward your feet. Once your hips, knees, and shoulders are in a straight line, return to the start position. Perform this exercise 10 times.

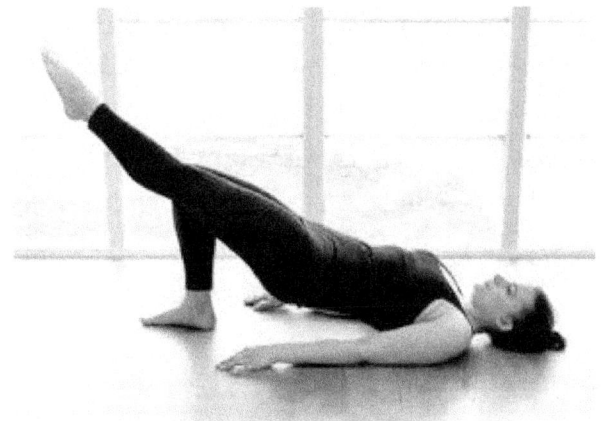

- Spine Stretch – This exercise is one of the simplest basic Pilates exercises. It focuses on your abs and emphasizes on increasing flexibility of your spine. Unlike the previous exercises, start this move by sitting with your legs apart and extended. Your hands should be on the mat between them. Keep your feet flexed as you push the upper body forward, circling your back while pulling your abs in and up. Inhale while rounding your back. Exhale while you roll back in a slow move, alternating 1 vertebra with the other. This exercise should be performed in 10 repetitions.

- The Pilates Curl – Start this exercise by lying on the mat, face towards the ceiling. Breathe out as you tilt your chin towards your chest. Do this movement by bringing your shoulders off the mat. Hold for one count and lower your back down in a slow manner. Make sure to focus on rising from the breastbone so that the abs will be engaged correctly. This would also avoid crunching your neck.

- The Crisscross – Start this exercise by facing up on the mat while your hands are behind your neck. Your elbows should be wide. Raise your head, neck, and shoulders from the mat. Extend your left leg to a high diagonal while your right leg reaches your left armpit.

Alternate the movement between two legs.

- The Double Straight Leg Stretch – Start this exercise with your back flat on the mat, face up. Your palms should be at the back of your neck for support while your legs are bent towards your chest. Breathe out as your upper torso is brought off the mat. Extend your legs and keep your toes pointed towards the ceiling. Bring your legs to a 45-degree angle in 3 counts. Lift again for another count.

- Obliques – This exercise puts emphasis on strengthening abdominals as well as toning the waist. You can start this exercise by sitting up while legs apart. Raise your arms over your head. Breathe in and out as you turn to your side. Make sure your hip muscle guides you in this move. Breathe in while your arms are stretched out but keep hips still. Exhale and return to start position. This exercise is performed in 4 sets.

- Shoulder Bridge – This exercise puts emphasis on the abs and back. You can start this exercise by lying flat on your back. Keep feet apart equal to the width of your hip. Arms should be on your sides. Raise hips with your back in place. The muscles in your hamstrings should be engaged while your buttocks stay tight to hold position in 5 counts. Lower yourself to the surface in a slow move.

- Letter "T" – This exercise puts emphasis on your back muscles. You can start this exercise with your stomach flat on the mat, feet together. Raise your arms slightly as you lift your chest off the mat. Bring your hands out, palms faced down for balance. Make sure your hands and palms are perpendicular to your body. Breathe in and out while you move arms behind in parallel with your back. Keep your waist down on the mat using your back muscles to keep them close to your body.

- Kneeling Side Kicks – This exercise puts emphasis on toning the buttocks and thighs. Start this exercise in kneeling position. Lean towards your left while your left hand stays on the mat under your shoulder. Your right hand should be behind your head, elbows pointed outwards. Your right leg should be parallel to the floor. Make sure your torso is still. Start kicking to your front and back. Repeat movement 5 times for each leg.

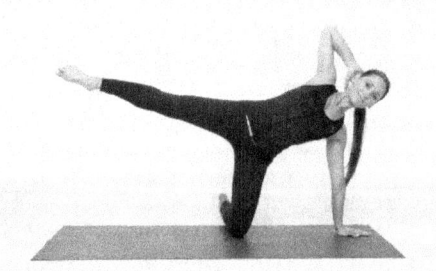

- Leg Swings – This exercise puts emphasis on raising heart rate and toning the legs. Start this exercise by standing straight, arms across the chest parallel to the height of your shoulders. Engage your abs as you exhale. Raise your right knee towards your right elbow. In an abrupt manner, lower your right leg. Repeat movement on the left side. Switch sides at least 10 times.

Chapter 7- How To Stay Motivated.

I want to start this chapter by taking about how you can stay motivated when you are doing Pilates. All the information in the world is not going to do you any good if you are not motivated to put it into use or if you lose your motivation after just a few days so I want to go over a few ways you can stay motivated and not quit.

The first tip I have for you, I referred to earlier and it is creating a calendar. On this calendar you are going to schedule your work outs, you will need to get a red and a green fine tipped marker because you are going to put a green X on the days that you actually work out and a red X on the days you do not. What you will find is you will have three or four green X's in a row and you will not want to put a red X on your calendar, you will associate this with failure which of course no one wants in their life. You will have days that you will work out simply because you do not want to put a red X on your calendar.

The next thing you can do is find someone to be accountable to, this can be your husband, best friend or even those on social networking. Each day you work out, you will be able to say you did it, you took the time and you put yourself before anything else in life, you are making changes in your life. If you don't exercise you have to let them know that as well and we all know we never want to admit to someone else that we have not followed through with our commitments, the thing you have to do is be honest. It is very easy to lie and say oh yeah I worked out but you need to remember in a month when you are not showing any results, they are going to know you lied.

Many people will say that as long as they are seeing results they will stay motivated. You may think this at first and you may think that losing weight quickly is going to make you want to exercise each day, but what happens when you are tired or you get sick or you just don't make the time for Pilates in your life? You miss a day, it turns into two, suddenly it is a month later and you have not worked out. You have stopped your diet, you're not drinking the correct amount of water your body needs and you are back to square one. Yes you are going to see results that is a given, if you follow what I have told you in this book, you are going to see results that is not going to be enough to keep you motivated because after a few weeks it is natural for people to start losing their motivation.

You need to change your perspective. This was extremely important for me in my early days. You see I work a lot, I am a single mother with three children and one who suffers from disabilities, my children are home schooled, I rescue dogs and I have a large farm to care for. I kept telling myself I didn't have the time there was no way I could take 30 minutes out of each day to exercise. Then I realized that I was spending about an hour and a half at night watching television, I was surfing the net for about an hour a day and often when I went to bed I would watch Netflix on my computer until I fell asleep. These all hit me as I was doing them and the thought would come, you could be exercising.

I began to see the light at that point but then I came up with another excuse, I'm tired. Trust me I get tired, we all do. We expect to be able to abuse our bodies, not provide proper nutrition or hydration for them and expect them to work at optimal levels. We can't figure out why we have no energy, why we can't accomplish the same things that others can, this causes depression and it is a vicious cycle. What had to click in my head was that I was very young, and I was living like an old woman, I had let having three children change my perspective of my body and accepted it as it was. I had to understand that taking care of me was going to increase my energy and it was going to make me feel better.

And finally there was one more thing I had to change my prospective on and that was the cost of healthy foods. I have already explained how people believe that healthy foods are more expensive and how that is not true. It took me a long time to learn how to eat healthy and even to this day I learn more all the time. It also took me a long time to understand serving sizes as well as how much I should be eating compared to what I was eating.

After I got my prospective changed, I knew I had to start focusing more on taking care of myself and what finally pushed me over the edge was that I would not just be exercising to be healthy but I would be teaching my children healthy habits that I never learned as a child. When you break it down like this, it is hard to not stay motivated.

Next you should set goals. Start with small ones, like doing Pilates for 10 minutes per day during week one. On week 2 your goal could be to do Pilates for 10 minutes per day and drink one gallon of water per day. On week three you could set your goal to doing Pilates for 10 minutes per day, drinking a gallon of water per day and eating a healthy breakfast each day. Do you see how each week we are keeping up with the goals of the previous week and simply adding on to them? It is best not to try and do all of this at the same time because as I discussed earlier if you change too much at one time you are going to become overwhelmed and none of it is going to stick.

You need to set a regular workout time. Just saying oh I will find the time to workout today is not going to cut it. You will not find the time, you will find reasons why you do not have time to exercise. I find that the morning is the best time to do Pilates, after you have woken up you can drink your water, slip into your workout clothing and start warming up go right into your workout, cool down and jump in the shower ready to start your day. After you have showered your body will be ready to eat without causing any cramps or upset from eating too soon after working out. You may have to wake up earlier and I already told you that it may seem impossible when you are tired but if you have to force yourself out of the bed at five in the morning like I do just so you can do your Pilates routine before you start your day that is what you will have to do. It will get easier with time, you will find that you jump out of bed ready to exercise after just a few weeks.

Vary the work out. If you look back to where I discussed what my normal workout week looks like you will see that never did I do the same work out two days in a row. You have to keep some variety in your workout routine but still keep it easy enough so you are not having to learn new exercises each day. If you want to do Pilates two days a week and light cardio two days a week and then go for a brisk walk two days a week that is completely fine set your routine up so that it works for you. You are still going to get the benefits of Pilates and you are going to program your body to work out each day. It will become as natural as breathing.

Keep a journal. Each evening before you go to bed write what challenges you encountered in your work out, whether it was struggling to get out of bed or even if it was struggling with making the correct food choices write it down. Write down how you felt after you worked out as well as after you made the right or wrong choice about what foods you would put in your body. Write down how much water you drank and how you feel about yourself reaching the goals you have set. Each week take a quick look back to see how far you have come, you will notice that you will have days where you are very motivated and days where you completely lack motivation but as time goes on you will see more days that you were motivated than not. This will also help you see what a difference not only doing Pilates, but eating right and staying hydrated is making in your life. This is a great motivator.

Now what are you supposed to do when your workouts become less of a challenge and more like a chore. You are not having fun when you are working out, it just seems like one more thing you have to do, you are not seeing the same results you were when you first started and you become frustrated. This is one place variety plays a very important role. At this point you are going to have to change up your routine possible moving on to more difficult work outs, if you are still working out for less than an hour per day you may need to increase your workout time as well.

Being consistent is my next tip for staying motivated. The more you do it, the better you will get and the more you will enjoy it. You will also see results much faster if you stick with it and are do your Pilates workouts on a regular basis. This is not to say that if you are sick in bed you need to do your work out but you need to make sure that as soon as you are better you are back at it.

Don't think of Pilates as a chore. You need to think of it the same way you would meditation or some other life changing practice you participate in. Pilates is not all about losing weight and gaining strength it is about bring balance to your body and your life. If you look at Pilates as nothing more than another work out, you will treat it like any other work out. You will stop doing it and it will just be one more program that did not work for you when the truth really is it is the program that could have worked for you had you stuck with it.

Understand that your body has natural imbalances and some that were caused from accidents. For example my left arm is much weaker than my right arm from an injury as a child as well as another as an adult. This is always going to be this way no matter how much I try to change it. Often times we just have to accept these little imbalances as unique qualities that make us who we are. This is not to say I do not work my left arm out just as much as my right arm, I just know my left arm will weaken faster and be sore after working out.

AND MORE...

Remember earlier when I told you that Pilates would help reduce stress? Next time you are trying to come up with a reason why you are too stressed out to exercise remember that after you spend just a few minutes doing Pilates you are going to feel so much better. I want to spend a few minutes talking about how Pilates can help to reduce stress and help you handle stress better.

Today the stress of life can seem unmanageable, we are always supposed to be somewhere doing something for someone, a kid is sick or we have projects overdue at work. Stress is not going anywhere and unless we do something about it, it is just going to get worse. This is where Pilates comes in. Pilates has been proven to help you deal with stress.

Pilates exercises are designed to work without tension, this means that although the muscles you are working during any particular exercise will be employed the rest of the body should remain as relaxed as possible. This helps the body to relax because you will only be engaging the particular muscles you need for each exercise.

Deep breathing has been proven to help reduce stress and Pilates focuses a lot of attention on deep breathing. Most of us are not breathing correctly and it is due to the stresses of life, Pilates will teach you how to breathe correctly this is called diaphragmatic breathing. It is focused breathing because most of the time we are so focused on the things going on around us that we forget to focus on how deep we are breathing which causes us to take short shallow breaths, practicing Pilates will retrain you to take focused deep breaths.

Your Pilates instructor will use imagery to help you reach a deep state of relaxation, much like imagery during relaxation hypnosis this is not day dreaming. The instructor will guide you into a peaceful state.

Pilates may seem like a completely foreign and odd exercise when you first start. There once was a time when people associated it with some type of false religion and there are those who even thought it was a form of satanic worshipping and all though it may seem different at first, you have to remember different doesn't mean bad. It is a wonderful way for you to change your life for the better, to feel better about yourself, to reduce stress, to lose weight and be a great example for your friends and family, and to balance your body. Given a few sessions it is almost guaranteed you will fall in love with it.

Pilates Myths

The first myth that I want to cover is that Pilates is too easy, this could not be further from the truth. If you believe that Pilates is too easy for you than try this. Get down in a push up position, not a girly push up but a real push up. Now push yourself up and hold for 1 minutes. Don't allow yourself to go back down like a regular push up. How easy was that? Pilates is not too easy for even the most athletic people. In fact it was tried by a very famous basketball player, he stated that after his first workout he was a little disappointed because he was not covered with sweat and was not hurting all over. He stuck with the program and six weeks later happily announced that he was stronger than he had ever been, he was in better shape than he had ever been and he owed it all to Pilates.

The next myth is that Pilates is a woman's work out. Now if you just read the above paragraph you will notice that I talked about a male basketball player. He loved Pilates but still many people think it is just for women. Up until recently most pictures of anyone doing Pilates was a woman with her legs extended above her head, most men would look at that picture and say no way. The truth is that Joseph Pilates actually designed his exercises with men in mind. The exercises were hard and although he did have some female clients he designed these exercises specifically for men to build up their bodies.

Only rich people do Pilates. This one is a little harder to debunk because private Pilates classes do cost a lot but this book is focused toward those who will be doing Pilates at home. If you are worried about someone judging you because you do Pilates simply don't tell them and you may want to consider if they should really be someone in your social group. You cannot judge a specific activity because certain people enjoy it. As long as you do not feel like you are acting stuck up or snobbish because you practice Pilates it should not matter who else practices it. For example let's look at kick boxing, there are many celebrities who have taken up kick boxing, does that mean it is only for the rich? No of course not, it means these people see the benefits of practicing kick boxing and were smart enough to give it a try. If you are looking for deals on Pilates training outside of your home, you can always watch for new gym openings, or when they offer a new class they usually have some type of deal. With the internet there really are deals to be had daily so you should not have an issue finding one.

I'm gonna be a supermodel....A lot of people think they are going to get amazing results in just a few work outs, they think they are going to have the body of a supermodel in a very short time. If that were true there would be a lot of Pilates instructors that were very very rich. The truth is, that it is going to help you lose weight, it is going to help you build muscle and with time you will have the body you dream of. Notice I said with time. Nothing happens overnight and that is just as true for Pilates as it is for any other work out. The results you see will depend on the work you put into it.

I will get a long lean body. Pilates is a great work out and it is going to help you reach your goals but if you are five foot two and your goal is to be five foot five, sorry Pilates is not going to help. Your body is only going to be as long as it is and there is nothing Pilates can do about that. What Pilates can do is give the illusion that you have a longer body. You see when you are overweight, your body can look squashed like someone put their hand on your head and pushed down. When you lose weight you will not look that way any longer, you will look longer than you did when you were overweight. Don't set your standards too high when it comes to having a long body, accept that you can look long and lean as long as you are willing to put in the work and you will be happy with the results.

Anyone can teach Pilates. As sad as it is to say this statement is true. Anyone can claim that they are a Pilates .instructor because at this point there are currently no regulations regarding Pilates instructors at this time. That does not mean that everyone teaching it knows what they are doing. You need to be very careful when you are searching for an instructor ask plenty of questions. In order to teach Pilates, you only have to take a weekend of training. This should be followed by many hours as a student. This is one reason I prefer finding my videos online instead of purchasing a DVD. It does not take much for a person to create a DVD and put it out for sale but when a persons reputation online is dependent upon the service they offer they are much more likely to provide you with information that is correct. And of course if you have issues you are always able to contact them via their website. If you are searching for online videos, you need to pay attention to the comments on the videos or blog. These are going to tell you if the person is real or not. You do need to watch for too many positive reviews with no questions because chances are those reviews were paid for.

The next myth is that Pilates will not help you lose weight. First of all if you are not exercising, adding any exercise into your life is going to help you lose weight. Pilates will help you lose weight but if you look at my one week of working out that I provided previously you will see that I do have aerobic workouts on my schedule. You see, you will burn calories while using Pilates but you are not going to burn as many calories as you would if you were doing aerobic exercises. But even if you do not want to add aerobic exercises you will be okay because Pilates is known for creating long lean muscles, the more muscles you have the more calories you will burn therefore as long as you do not take in more calories than you are burning you will be okay.

You should understand that generally Pilates is not used as a calorie burning exercise but a 150 pound person can burn 286 calories per hour of Pilates workouts. What makes people experience such a significant weigh loss with Pilates is that they are building lean muscle, increasing the amount of water they drink and changing the way they eat. It will strengthen your muscles so that you will be able to endure longer aerobic workouts, it will help with breathing so you do not get winded quickly when doing aerobic exercises, and it will help you to correct your posture which will help you look slimmer almost immediately.

Chapter 8: Getting The Most Out Of Your Pilates Workout.

To start off with I would like to talk a little bit about meditation. Even Pilates instructors who have been practicing Pilates for years and then try meditation are amazed at the results. You will do your normal morning workout with Pilates then in the evening before you go to bed you will spend some time meditating. You see Pilates has a lot to do with focusing on your breathing and imagery, meditation does as well, the more you meditate the easier it will be for you to focus during your Pilates work outs. Meditation also helps with sleep which will ensure you are getting enough rest before your next big work out. You can also use visualization to help motivate you when you meditate at night. You can spend some time visualizing yourself working out the next morning, you can visualize the results you want to see down the road. Visualize yourself being successful and when you feel like giving up you will have that image in your head.

If you really want to get the most out of your Pilates work out, you need to make sure you follow a healthy diet like the one I mentioned earlier in this book. You also need to make sure you are getting enough water. If you are already working out than adding Pilates will ensure you get the most out of all of the work outs you do.

What type of exercise do you need to be doing each week. Joseph Pilates suggested that you should use Pilates four times per week. You can start out with 10 minutes per day, it is recommended that you get 150 minutes of aerobic exercise each week as well so one and one half hours. I break this down to 30 minutes sections three times per week. And you should do some form of strength training for at least 30 minutes twice a week. Now this may seem like a lot so if you are just starting out don't let it overwhelm you. Only look at this as a point to work up to.

You also don't have to worry about purchasing or storing a bunch of weights, just look for videos for strength training without weights. You can find these for free online and you can find tons of aerobic videos online as well. Once you work up to this you should be spending about one hour per day total including warm ups and cool downs. Doing these other workouts is how you are going to get the best benefits from Pilates. You can also look online for a website that provides videos for all of these workouts. I have been able to find some that provided not only a workout calendar but they videos of all of the workouts for each day. This is the best type of program you can look for because they will start you off at a beginners level and you will work your way up to a more advanced level. This is also going to ensure you tone your body, lose weight and strengthen your muscles all at the same time.

You need to remember when you first start that nothing is easy when you are first learning it. This goes for everything in life including Pilates. What you have to remind yourself of is that it will get easier with time. Even when your muscles are sore and your body feels tired stick with the program remember why you chose to add Pilates to your exercise routine and push through.

You usually won't feel anything after you complete a Pilates work out, your muscles won't feel sore and you probably won't even sweat. You will start to feel it the next day this is why I recommend doing Pilates every other day and filling in with other work outs.

For example if you do Pilates on Monday, Wednesday and Friday (remember you will take Sunday off) You should focus on different exercises such as aerobics and strength training on Tuesday, Thursday and Saturday. You will work out a program that covers your needs, if you look at mine you will see I often do Pilates and a short aerobic workout on the same day. The next day I will focus on my arms, thighs or another part of my body. This is very important, you have to make sure you are not overworking your muscles. If your muscles are sore, let them rest and pick another set of muscles to work out.

Pilates is not for the body builder. Pilates creates lean muscle without bulking up. You can still lift weights, you can still do aerobic exercises but you will not be creating bulky muscles you will be creating lean muscles which is great if you are a woman! I spent my life working out and lifting weights, I didn't really see a problem with it until I was at work one day with a short sleeve shirt on, a guy was smoking and one of his ashes landed on my arm which caused my arm to flex. I will never forget the reaction of that guy. Most people would be flattered but as a woman who really wants to be seen as feminine and not a muscle woman it upset me. The next weekend I was out on a date and raised my arms up to put my hair back and the guy surprised said wow your arms are bigger than mine. That was my breaking point. I stopped lifting weights and thought there was no hope. My arms became weak and wimpy, I knew I had to find something to help and I found Pilates. Today I am thrilled with my arms, thrilled with my workout routine and thrilled with Pilates. I want to share it with everyone!

Not only did I find out how great it would be for my arms but I saw the results in my thighs as well. I again had very muscular thighs, they were strong but big and I honestly hated them because well they were just not what I wanted. With Pilates I have been able to keep the muscles without the bulk. Now my thighs are slim and I love them.

I am telling you all of this to show you that no matter what you are trying to accomplish you can do it with

Pilates. Let me tell you about a friend of mine. She was in her 50's and was extremely overweight. She always asked me for help with her weight but because she was so unhealthy I really didn't know what to do. Now this woman was so out of shape that she would spend her life sitting on her couch watching television. If she needed to sweep the floors to her house she became exhausted. She couldn't take the dog out to the front porch even. She was falling asleep sitting up and not sleeping at night.

I knew something had to be done so the first thing we changed was her amount of water intake. This is very important if you are overweight. Once I got her to start drinking more water we changed her diet. I did not do this gradually because as far as I am concerned when someone gets to this point their life is in danger and there is no time to waste.

Since she lived a very sedentary lifestyle I knew I could not start her out with aerobics and decided to give Pilates a shot with her. I started her out at 10 minutes per day 4 days per week. It was all she could do to do this much but she was able to do it. Her body was not sore and she learned that she was able to do more than just sit around all day. As the weeks went by, she learned that she could do more and that included cleaning her house, taking her dog out for a walk and adding aerobics into her workout program. She is now 160 pounds, still slightly overweight but much more active than when she began, she is on her way to the body and life she has always wanted. I watched this woman go from someone who thought everything was wrong with her and had no hope for the future is now unstoppable.

Maybe this woman reminds you of yourself, maybe you don't think you can work out but Pilates is the one workout that I can guarantee will work for you no matter what your limitations, no matter how out of shape you are, you can start using Pilates today and change your life just like my friend did.

I want to finish this book by talking about a few things you need to remember when you are beginning Pilates. The first thing is that no amount of Pilates is going to change the amount of food you eat and if you don't change the amount of food you eat you will not see the benefits from Pilates. I have stressed through the book the importance of changing your diet but I cannot stress it enough. If you do not change your eating habits and this incudes increasing the amount of water you are drinking you will find that you will basically be treading water. You will be trying as hard as you can when you are working out, you may even add in some aerobic exercised but you be losing minimal weight and building minimal muscles. Think of it like this. If you were going to build a house and someone brought you to build the house with. Every time it rained you had to start over and try again to build this house out of mud. This is basically what you are doing, you wake up early and exercise followed by a huge breakfast and a glass of soda, you eat whatever you want all day long. The food is like the rain, then the next day you are starting all over again never seeing any results. Now let's think about your car, it will run if you put cheap oil and cheap gas in it correct. It will do what it is supposed to do for a period of time and then you will start seeing problems if you on the other hand use premium gas and premium oils you will see that your car lasts much longer. The same goes for your body. The junk food is the cheap gas and oils, but healthy fruits, vegetables, meats and nuts are the premium gas.

When you are tempted to eat those foods you know are not good for you think about all of the time you put in to your workout, this can remind you that you really don't need that tub of ice cream.

The second thing you need to remember is that it takes time to learn the language. You are adjusting to an entirely different lifestyle and in a way you will be learning an entirely different language. This takes time and there is no reward for the person who finishes the fastest. Take your time. If you want to watch your Pilates video before you try it go ahead but don't let it overwhelm you, don't sit there and think there is no way you can do it. You never know until you try.

And that brings me to the third thing you need to remember. You will never see results if you don't stick it out. Even on the hard days when you don't feel like working out you need to remind yourself that skipping one day will lead to two and the next thing you know you have wasted a month and nothing has changed. Even if you have to force yourself just do it. It will be worth it all in the end.

You also need to remember that unlike many exercise and diet programs being promoted today, Pilates is not a fad. It is actually about 100 years old. Remember that Joseph Pilates started off as a very sickly child, he was prone to asthma attacks and was always getting sick so no matter what problems you may be having Pilates will help you. It is not a quick fix but with consistency you will see your symptoms fading and your body getting stronger.

Next, you need to remember that doing Pilates is not just working through the moves, it is focusing on each movement, it is about the precision and grace of each movement. The truth is anyone can perform these moves but if they are not done correctly they are not going to benefit the person doing them. It may seem difficult at first to focus on pulling your belly button in, breathing correctly, keeping the correct posture, and learning the exercise but as long as you continue to practice it will all come together for you. Remember that no matter what, when you do a bicep curl you are doing a bicep curl unless you are using Pilates in which case you are engaging your core before you do the bicep curl. This is what makes Pilates different from any other exercise.

Finally I want to remind you that although many people believe that Pilates is just for the abs, it really is a full body work out. Yes you will be engaging your abs a lot and you will get a flat stomach much faster when you use Pilates than you will any other form of exercise but Pilates is so much more than just an ab work out. You are going to learn how to bring your mind and your body together to work as one for your benefit, you are going to engage each set of your muscles throughout your entire body but keep your core engaged the entire work out. I guarantee the day after you do your first Pilates work out it will not just be your abs that are sore.

Pilates is great for everyone who is willing to put the time and effort in. I warn you that once many people get through their first few work outs and start seeing results they are hooked. Pilates can be that one thing that you use to change your life right now and in the future. Don't worry if you can't hold positions as long as the instructor on the video hold them as long as you can and the instructor should give you a positon you can work from if you are getting tired. Each day you will see that you can hold the positions longer and longer and this means that you are building and strengthening your muscles. This means you are benefiting from Pilates!

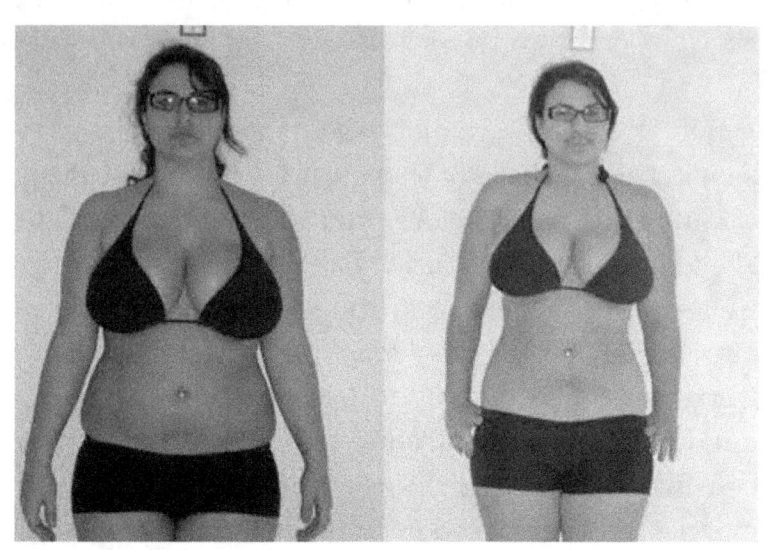

Conclusion

Thank you again for downloading this book!

I hope this book was able to help you gain more knowledge on the Pilates Method. The Pilates workout routine provided in this book is a full body workout that bestows many health benefits.

In this book, the Pilates workout routine is primarily designed for beginners although those who are veterans in Pilates can also carry out the exercises for added challenge.

Each exercise can be more difficult than the last as you go on with the series of exercises. As a beginner, you have the option of remaining on the first and/or second set of exercise created for the enhancement of the abdominals. That is, if you find the later movements too difficult. Beginners can repeat the movements that they are comfortable with until they achieve the proper form to do the exercises. Once you improve your strength, you can move on to a harder movement.

On the other hand, if you find the movements simple and can keep a proper from with each exercise, you can follow the entire routine and increase difficulty each time. In fact, you can even jump from one exercise to harder ones or double the repetitions for each movement.

The next step is to take the plunge and get into performing the Pilates moves you have learned. You will not regret anything as Pilates promises improved mental and physical well-being.

It also integrates your mind and body through its main principles: complete focus, concentration, and breathing. Thus, Pilates is a great method in order to connect with you self, find peace, and reduce levels of stress.

The key to a successful Pilates workout routine is modification. Every exercise involved in Pilates has been developed and modified for a safe yet challenging workout for individuals at a given level (beginner, intermediate, and advanced).

Pilates comprises a set of easy exercises, which involve basic movement principles from which Pilates has been founded. Pilates is also referred to as a method of functional fitness given that its principles emphasize having better posture as well as efficient and graceful movements.

Finally, if you enjoyed this book, please take the time to share your thoughts and post a review on Amazon. It'd be greatly appreciated!

Thank you and good luck!

Check Out My Other Books

Below you'll find some of my other popular books that are popular on Amazon and Kindle as well. Simply click on the links below to check them out. Alternatively, you can visit my author page on Amazon to see other work done by me.

http://www.amazon.com/NrBooks/e/B00ET2BG9Y/

If the links do not work, for whatever reason, you can simply search for these titles on the Amazon website to find them.

www.ingramcontent.com/pod-product-compliance
Lightning Source LLC
Chambersburg PA
CBHW060428290526
45791CB00002B/897